Skinny
Cocktails

The only guide you'll ever need to go out, have fun, and still fit into your skinny jeans

JACLYN WILSON FOLEY & RAY FOLEY

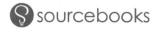 sourcebooks

Published by Sourcebooks, Inc.
P.O. Box 4410, Naperville, Illinois 60567–4410
(630) 961–3900
Fax: (630) 961–2168
www.sourcebooks.com

Library of Congress Cataloging-in-Publication Data

Foley, Jaclyn.
  Skinny cocktails / Jaclyn Wilson Foley and Ray Foley.
      p. cm.
  Includes index.
  1. Cocktails. 2. Reducing diets—Recipes. I. Foley, Ray. II. Title.
  TX951.F583 2010
  641.8'74—dc22

                              2010035794

Printed and bound in Canada.
WC 10 9 8 7 6 5

Contents

Acknowledgments

To the great people who work at Sourcebooks, especially Sara Kase, who has been a great help with both *Girls' Night* and this book.

To Lauren Saccone, for her help always and for being Lauren Saccone.

To all the readers of *Bartender Magazine* and www.bartender.com.

Special thanks to Terri Nelson, Martha Levy, David Mandler from the Susan Magrino Agency in New York and Stolichnaya Vodka, Lynette Setlich for Sunkist Foodservice, Allison Petschauer from Rose's Lime Juice, Alana Hadmin from Alison Brod Public Relations, Ali Smolens from Maury Rogoff PR & Marketing and paQui Tequila, the crew at Imperial Brands, Amanda Baiada from Ocean Spray, Rebekah Polster from Gregory White PR,

Peggy McCormick from MMM Marketing for Dole Foodservice, Mary Sullivan from Deussen Global Communications, Jaclyn Sisbarro from 5W Public Relations and Three Olives Vodka and 1800 Tequila, Cecilia Mena from FORMULATIN and Herradura Tequila, Erin Jevis from Bulldog Gin, Page Jeter from Entertainment Fusion Group and TY KU Liqueur, Annelies Brandes, Tanya Thomas from Truth B Told and Corzo Tequila, Karlyn Monroe from Rémy Cointreau USA, and all the major liquor companies that have supported *Bartender Magazine* and helped to support this book.

Drink healthy, drink wise, drink responsibly, and never ever drink and drive.

Welcome to the Skinny Life

Ever had a Long Island iced tea and wondered why you couldn't button your pants the next day? It's because you drank an extra 700 calories—and that's if you had only one drink! It happens to the best of us. We know a glass of wine won't do much damage, but when everyone at the table is ordering frosty beers…well, what do you think happens? We obviously get drink envy and go for it. And sometimes on the first gorgeous day of the season, the only thing that will hit the spot is a blended strawberry margarita. Or a mojito. Or a flirty cocktail. You get the picture.

Everyone likes to let loose and have a drink sometimes, but no one wants that drink to go right to their thighs. Even so, whether you're planning on kicking back after a hectic day or vamping it up for a night out, the last thing you want to do is obsess about calories. Tell me you haven't been here and I'll be shocked: "How many calories are in this drink? Can I have more than one? Will I be able to go to the beach tomorrow and not be mistaken for a distant relative of Shamu?" Talk about a buzz kill.

Enter *Skinny Cocktails*, a woman's must-have cocktail companion. Including no-fear recipes, easy-access calorie counts, and minimal-damage mixers, this will be your dream guide to a stress-free skinny life. And lucky for you, this book is probably small enough to fit in your purse. Maybe not in your tiny clutch, but you can't fool me. I know you own more than one bag, sistah. With *Skinny Cocktails* you can be trim *and* toasted. Skinny and sauced. Beautiful and belligerent. Well, maybe we don't want to get belligerent. Let's keep it classy, ladies.

Written by the publishers of number one industry insider *Bartender Magazine*, this book is a must-have for calorie-conscious women like you who still want to enjoy the drinks they love. After all, you shouldn't have to lose the glamour of having a few cocktails with your girls for anything. With a little consideration before you booze, the top bartenders in America will teach you that making drinks (and slyly keeping track of calories) can be as satisfying and effortless as slipping on your Little Black Dress.

So put on your skinny jeans, call your girlfriends, shake up some cocktails…and get ready for your best night out yet!

Drink Tools:
Getting Ready to Get
Your Skinny On

You'll need the proper tools to create outstanding drinks. Below are a few that will help make you a pro. These tools are just suggestions, but if you have a well-stocked bar, it will be easier to create the drinks throughout this book. And you'll be able to make 'em in less time, too.

Bar Spoon: A long spoon for stirring cocktails or pitchers.

Blender: Used for blending drinks or crushing ice. Save your blade by always pouring in the liquid before the ice.

Cocktail Shaker and Mixing/Measuring Glass: There are countless designs to choose from, but the standard is the Boston shaker. It's a mixing glass that fits snuggly into a stainless steel cone.

Commercial Juicer: The Sunkist brand commercial juicer can endure extended daily usage, extracting between 10–12 gallons of juice per hour using precut citrus. Its unique oscillating strainer helps separate the juice from the pulp.

Ice Bag: To crush ice use a rubber mallet and a lint-free or canvas ice bag, often referred to as a Lewis Ice Bag.

Ice Bucket: Should have a vacuum seal and the capacity to hold three trays of ice.

Ice Scoop/Tongs/Ice Pick: Never use your hands to pick up ice. Use a scoop or tongs. The ice pick can help you separate ice or break it up.

Jigger/Measuring Glass: Glass or metal, all drinks should be made using these bar tools. Remember that drinks on the rocks and mixed drinks should contain no more than 2 oz. of alcohol.

Knife and Cutting Board: A sturdy board and a small, very sharp paring knife are essential to cutting fruit garnishes.

Muddler: Use this small wooden bat or pestle to crush fruit, herbs, or cracked ice. Muddlers come in all different sizes.

Napkins/Coasters: To place a drink on, hold a drink with, and for basic convenience.

Pitcher of Water: Keep it clean. Someone always wants water, and you certainly will use it.

Pourer: A helpful way to pour directly into the glass. A lidded spout helps keep everything but the drink out.

Stirrers/Straws: Use them to sip, stir, and mix drinks. Glass is preferred for mixing and stirring.

Strainer: The strainer, quite simply, prevents ice from pouring out of the shaker. The two most common types in use are the Hawthorne and the Julep. The Hawthorne, with its distinctive coil rim, is most often used when pouring from the metal part of the Boston shaker. The Julep is a perforated metal spoon like a strainer and is used when pouring from the glass part of the Boston shaker.

Wine Bottle/Opener: They come in all shapes and sizes, but the best is the industry standard waiter's opener. It has a sharp blade to open cans and can also be used to snap off bottle tops.

Part I
Calories and Carbohydrates

Not all liquors, beers, and mixers are created
equal. Some are lower in calories, some in
carbohydrates. Following are lists of common liquid
indulgences to help you get a grip on your options.

Calories and Carbohydrates
for Liquors

All amounts are per 1 oz.

Top 10 Low-Calorie Liquors

10. Captain Morgan Silver spiced rum (70 proof)
    61 calories
9. Captain Morgan Original spiced rum
   (70 proof)
   58 calories
8. Malibu rum flavored with fruit essence
   57 calories
7. Gordon's citrus vodka
   56 calories
6. Gordon's orange vodka
   55 calories
5. Gordon's Wildberry vodka
   49 calories
4. Port
   46 calories

3. Captain Morgan Parrot Bay Sunset Surf tropical malt beverage
   21 calories
2. Captain Morgan Parrot Bay Wave Runner tropical malt beverage
   21 calories
1. Captain Morgan Parrot Bay Matava Blue tropical malt beverage
   19 calories

Zero-Carb Liquors

Bourbon whiskey (80 proof)
Brandy (80 proof)
Brandy (86 proof)
Brandy (100 proof)
Buchanan's whisky
Bulleit bourbon
Bulloch Lade scotch whisky
Captain Morgan Original spiced rum (70 proof)
Cîroc vodka
Cognac (80 proof)
Cognac (86 proof)
Cognac (100 proof)

Crème de menthe (72 proof)
Crown Royal whisky
Crown Royal Special Reserve whisky
Don Julio tequila
George Dickel No. 12 whisky
George Dickel No. 8 whisky
Gin (80 proof)
Gin (86 proof)
Gin (90 proof)
Gin (100 proof)
Gordon's citrus vodka
Johnnie Walker Black whisky
Johnnie Walker Blue whisky
Johnnie Walker Gold whisky
Johnnie Walker Red whisky
Lagavulin whisky
Malibu rum (48 proof)
Myers's Legend rum
Myers's Original dark rum
Myers's Platinum white rum
Oban whisky
Ron Añejo rum
Rum (80 proof)
Rum (86 proof)
Rum (90 proof)
Rum (100 proof)

Seagram's 7 Crown whisky
Seagram's V.O. Gold whisky
Seagram's V.O. whisky
Sobieski vodka
Talisker whisky
Tanqueray gin
Tanqueray gin, No. Ten
Tanqueray Sterling citrus vodka
Tanqueray Sterling vodka
Tequila (80 proof)
Usher's scotch whisky
Vodka (80 proof)
Vodka (86 proof)
Vodka (90 proof)
Vodka (100 proof)
Whisky, Scotch (80 proof)
Whisky, Scotch (86 proof)
Whisky, Scotch (90 proof)
Whisky, Scotch (100 proof)

99 schnapps
99 calories   •   5g carbs

Bols Advocaat liqueur
85 calories   •   9g carbs

Bols apricot brandy
87 calories • 9g carbs

Bols butterscotch schnapps
72 calories • 11g carbs

Bols cherry brandy
78 calories • 9g carbs

Bols coconut liqueur
103 calories • 11g carbs

Bols crème de bananes
96 calories • 11g carbs

Bols dark crème de cacao
100 calories • 15g carbs

Bols Gold Strike cinnamon liqueur
103 calories • 11g carbs

Bols green crème de menthe
120 calories • 14g carbs

Bols green curaçao liqueur
72 calories • 7g carbs

Bols kiwi liqueur
103 calories • 11g carbs

Bols Kontiki red orange liqueur
103 calories • 11g carbs

Bols melon liqueur
103 calories • 11g carbs

Bols orange liqueur
103 calories • 11g carbs

Bols orange curaçao liqueur
72 calories • 7g carbs

Bols peach liqueur
103 calories • 11g carbs

Bols peppermint liqueur
103 calories • 11g carbs

Bols Pumpkin Smash liqueur
103 calories • 11g carbs

Bols triple sec
103 calories • 11g carbs

Bols white crème de cacao
100 calories • 15g carbs

Bourbon whiskey (80 proof)
66 calories • 0g carbs

Brandy (80 proof)
64 calories • 0g carbs

Brandy (86 proof)
70 calories • 0g carbs

Brandy (100 proof)
82 calories • 0g carbs

Buchanan's whisky
64 calories • 0g carbs

Bulleit bourbon
72 calories • 0g carbs

Bulloch Lade scotch whisky
64 calories • 0g carbs

Captain Morgan Original spiced rum (70 proof)
58 calories • 0g carbs

Captain Morgan Parrot Bay coconut rum
    62 calories • 7g carbs

Captain Morgan Parrot Bay Matava Blue tropical malt beverage
    19 calories • 3g carbs

Captain Morgan Parrot Bay passion fruit rum
    63 calories • 7g carbs

Captain Morgan Parrot Bay Sunset Surf tropical malt beverage
    21 calories • 3g carbs

Captain Morgan Parrot Bay Wave Runner tropical malt beverage
    21 calories • 3g carbs

Captain Morgan Private Stock rum
    73 calories • 3g carbs

Captain Morgan Silver spiced rum (70 proof)
    61 calories • 1g carbs

Cîroc vodka
    64 calories • 0g carbs

Coffee liqueur (53 proof)
95 calories • 13g carbs

Coffee liqueur (63 proof)
87 calories • 9g carbs

Coffee liqueur with cream (34 proof)
93 calories • 6g carbs

Cognac (80 proof)
64 calories • 0g carbs

Cognac (86 proof)
70 calories • 0g carbs

Cognac (100 proof)
82 calories • 0g carbs

Crème de menthe (72 proof)
105 calories • 0g carbs

Crown Royal whisky
64 calories • 0g carbs

Crown Royal Special Reserve whisky
64 calories • 0g carbs

DeKuyper amaretto almond liqueur
   110 calories • 17g carbs

DeKuyper Apple Barrel schnapps
   72 calories • 8g carbs

DeKuyper blueberry schnapps
   72 calories • 11g carbs

DeKuyper blue curaçao liqueur
   72 calories • 7g carbs

DeKuyper Buttershots liqueur
   72 calories • 11g carbs

DeKuyper cactus juice schnapps
   103 calories • 11g carbs

DeKuyper Cheri-Beri Pucker schnapps
   103 calories • 11g carbs

DeKuyper cherry brandy
   78 calories • 9g carbs

DeKuyper coffee liqueur
   103 calories • 11g carbs

DeKuyper crème de bananes
96 calories • 11g carbs

DeKuyper dark crème de cacao
100 calories • 15g carbs

DeKuyper Grape Pucker schnapps
72 calories • 11g carbs

DeKuyper Harvest Pear
103 calories • 11g carbs

DeKuyper hazelnut liqueur
103 calories • 11g carbs

DeKuyper Hot Damn cinnamon schnapps
103 calories • 11g carbs

DeKuyper Island Blue Pucker schnapps
72 calories • 11g carbs

DeKuyper Key Largo schnapps
72 calories • 11g carbs

DeKuyper Mad Melon schnapps
72 calories • 11g carbs

DeKuyper Marasquin cherry liqueur
73 calories • 9g carbs

DeKuyper Peachtree schnapps
72 calories • 7g carbs

DeKuyper peppermint schnapps
83 calories • 7 1/2g carbs

DeKuyper Pucker Strawberry Passion schnapps
72 calories • 9g carbs

DeKuyper Raspberry Pucker schnapps
72 calories • 11g carbs

DeKuyper Razzmatazz liqueur
72 calories • 11g carbs

DeKuyper Sour Apple Pucker schnapps
72 calories • 8g carbs

DeKuyper Sour Peach Pucker schnapps
72 calories • 7g carbs

DeKuyper Sour Watermelon Pucker schnapps
72 calories • 11g carbs

DeKuyper strawberry liqueur
103 calories • 11g carbs

DeKuyper triple sec
103 calories • 11g carbs

DeKuyper Wildberry schnapps
103 calories • 11g carbs

Don Julio tequila
64 calories • 0g carbs

George Dickel No. 12 whisky
72 calories • 0g carbs

George Dickel No. 8 whisky
64 calories • 0g carbs

Gin (80 proof)
64 calories • 0g carbs

Gin (86 proof)
70 calories • 0g carbs

Gin (90 proof)
73 calories • 0g carbs

Gin (100 proof)
82 calories • 0g carbs

Goldschläger cinnamon schnapps
99 calories • 7g carbs

Gordon's citrus vodka
56 calories • 0g carbs

Gordon's orange vodka
55 calories • 2g carbs

Gordon's Wildberry vodka
49 calories • 1g carbs

Johnnie Walker Black whisky
64 calories • 0g carbs

Johnnie Walker Blue whisky
64 calories • 0g carbs

Johnnie Walker Gold whisky
64 calories • 0g carbs

Johnnie Walker Red whisky
64 calories • 0g carbs

Lagavulin whisky
    69 calories • 0g carbs

Malibu rum (48 proof)
    68 calories • 0g carbs

Malibu rum flavored with fruit essence
    57 calories • 6g carbs

Myers's Legend rum
    64 calories • 0g carbs

Myers's Original dark rum
    64 calories • 0g carbs

Myers's Platinum white rum
    64 calories • 0g carbs

Oban whisky
    70 calories • 0g carbs

Port
    46 calories • 3 1/2g carbs

Ron Añejo rum
    64 calories • 0g carbs

Rum (80 proof)
    64 calories   •   0g carbs

Rum (86 proof)
    70 calories   •   0g carbs

Rum (90 proof)
    73 calories   •   0g carbs

Rum (100 proof)
    82 calories   •   0g carbs

Rumpleminze schnapps
    113 calories   •   9g carbs

Seagram's 7 Crown whisky
    64 calories   •   0g carbs

Seagram's V.O. Gold whisky
    64 calories   •   0g carbs

Seagram's V.O. whisky
    64 calories   •   0g carbs

Sobieski vodka
    100 calories   •   0g carbs

Talisker whisky
73 calories • 0g carbs

Tanqueray gin
76 calories • 0g carbs

Tanqueray gin, No. Ten
75 calories • 0g carbs

Tanqueray Sterling citrus vodka
64 calories • 0g carbs

Tanqueray Sterling vodka
64 calories • 0g carbs

Tequila (80 proof)
64 calories • 0g carbs

Vodka (80 proof)
73 calories • 0g carbs

Vodka (86 proof)
70 calories • 0g carbs

Vodka (90 proof)
73 calories • 0g carbs

Vodka (100 proof)
   82 calories • 0g carbs

Whisky, Scotch (80 proof)
   73 calories • 0g carbs

Whisky, Scotch (86 proof)
   70 calories • 0g carbs

Whisky, Scotch (90 proof)
   73 calories • 0g carbs

Whisky, Scotch (100 proof)
   82 calories • 0g carbs

Calories and Carbohydrates
for Beer

All amounts are per 12 oz. bottle.

Beers under 100 Calories

Beck's Premier Light
  64 calories
Budweiser Select
  99 calories
Budweiser Select 55
  55 calories
Busch Light
  95 calories
Heineken Premium Light
  99 calories
Michelob Ultra
  95 calories
Michelob Ultra Light
  73 calories
Miller Genuine Draft Light 64 (MGD 64)
  64 calories

Miller Light
   96 calories
Yuengling Light
   90 calories
Yuengling Light Lager
   99 calories

Beck's Dark
   142 calories   •   10g carbs

Beck's Pilsner
   138 calories   •   9g carbs

Beck's Premier Light
   64 calories   •   4g carbs

Blue Moon Ale
   228 calories   •   18g carbs

Bud Dry
   130 calories   •   8g carbs

Bud Light
   110 calories   •   6 1/2g carbs

Budweiser

145 calories • 11g carbs

Budweiser Select

99 calories • 3g carbs

Budweiser Select 55

55 calories • 0g carbs

Busch

133 calories • 10g carbs

Busch Light

95 calories • 3g carbs

Coors Light

102 calories • 7g carbs

Coors Original

192 calories • 14g carbs

Corona Extra

148 calories • 14g carbs

Corona Light

105 calories • 5g carbs

Dos Equis XX Amber

146 calories • 12g carbs

Dos Equis XX Lager

142 calories • 11g carbs

Guinness Draught

126 calories • 10g carbs

Guinness Extra Stout

176 calories • 14g carbs

Heineken

150 calories • 12g carbs

Heineken Premium Light

99 calories • 7g carbs

Heineken Special Dark

175 calories • 16g carbs

Killian's Irish Red

163 calories • 15g carbs

Michelob Amber

110 calories • 4g carbs

Michelob Light
 123 calories • 9g carbs

Michelob Ultra
 95 calories • 3g carbs

Michelob Ultra Light
 73 calories • 2g carbs

Miller Genuine Draft
 143 calories • 13g carbs

Miller Genuine Draft Light
 110 calories • 7g carbs

Miller Genuine Draft Light 64 (MGD 64)
 64 calories • 0g carbs

Miller Light
 96 calories • 3g carbs

Newcastle Brown Ale
 140 calories • 13g carbs

Pabst Blue Ribbon
 113 calories • 8g carbs

Pabst Light
111 calories • 8g carbs

Red Stripe Jamaican Ale
153 calories • 14g carbs

Sam Adams Boston Lager
180 calories • 19g carbs

Sam Adams Light
119 calories • 10g carbs

Sapporo Light
119 calories • 9g carbs

Sierra Nevada Pale Bock
218 calories • 20g carbs

Sierra Nevada Porter
194 calories • 18g carbs

Sierra Nevada Stout
225 calories • 22g carbs

Sierra Nevada Wheat Ale
153 calories • 13g carbs

Stella Artois
154 calories • 12g carbs

Yuengling Black & Tan
135 calories • 14g carbs

Yuengling Light
90 calories • 7g carbs

Yuengling Light Lager
99 calories • 9g carbs

Yuengling Premium
120 calories • 12g carbs

Calories and Carbohydrates

for Champagne, Wine, and Mixers

10 Mixers under 10 Calories (per 1-oz. serving)

1. Lemon juice (fresh)—8 calories
2. Lime juice (fresh)—8 calories
3. V8 Splash Berry Blend—8 calories
4. Acerola juice (fresh)—6 calories
5. Carrot juice (fresh)—6 calories
6. V8 vegetable juice—6 calories
7. Tomato juice (canned)—5 calories
8. Red Bull (sugar free)—1 calorie
9. Club soda—0 calories
10. Diet cola—0 calories

Champagne
19 calories • 0g carbs

Sake
39 calories • 1 1/2g carbs

Wine (Red)
25 calories • 1g carbs

Wine (White)
24 calories • 1g carbs

Acerola juice (fresh)
6 calories • 1g carbs

Apple juice (canned or bottled)
13 calories • 3 1/2g carbs

Blackberry juice (canned)
11 calories • 2g carbs

Carrot juice (canned)
11 calories • 3g carbs

Carrot juice (fresh)
6 calories • 1 1/2g carbs

Cherry cola
   13 calories   •   3 1/2g carbs

Club soda
   0 calories   •   0g carbs

Cola
   90 calories   •   3 1/2g carbs

Cola, caffeine-free
   12 calories   •   3 1/2g carbs

Cola, diet
   0 calories   •   0g carbs

Cola with lime
   12 calories   •   3 1/2g carbs

Cranberry cocktail
   17 calories   •   4 1/2g carbs

Ginger ale
   10 calories   •   2g carbs

Grape juice (bottled)
   18 calories   •   5g carbs

Grapefruit juice (fresh)
    12 calories • 3g carbs

Lemonade
    15 calories • 4g carbs

Lemon juice (fresh)
    8 calories • 3g carbs

Lemon-lime soda
    13 calories • 3g carbs

Lime juice (fresh)
    8 calories • 3g carbs

Orange juice (fresh)
    13 calories • 3g carbs

Orange juice concentrate (frozen)
    56 calories • 14g carbs

Orange soda
    15 calories • 4g carbs

Pineapple juice (canned or bottled)
    16 calories • 4 1/2g carbs

Pomegranate juice
15 calories • 4g carbs

Red Bull
13 calories • 3g carbs

Red Bull (sugar-free)
1 calorie • 0g carbs

Root beer
13 calories • 3g carbs

Tangerine juice (canned)
14 calories • 3g carbs

Tangerine juice (fresh)
12 calories • 3g carbs

Tomato juice (canned)
5 calories • 1g carbs

Tonic water
10 calories • 3g carbs

V8 vegetable juice
6 calories • 1g carbs

V8 Splash Berry Blend
8 calories • 2g carbs

Vanilla Coca-Cola
12 calories • 3 1/2g carbs

Part II
The Skinny Cocktails

Sure, you can concoct your own drink using the lists in part I. But you can also use a few extra ingredients, such as nectars, a scant amount of sugar, a splash of simple syrup, no-calorie sweetener, etc., to make the delicious cocktails listed below. All clock in at a respectable 200 calories or less, so let's get mixing!

5-0 Cosmo—*50 calories*
   3 oz. Ocean Spray diet cranberry juice drink
   3/4 oz. Absolut Raspberri vodka
   Squeeze lime
   Lime twist for garnish

   Shake over ice until cold. Strain into a chilled glass and garnish with the lime twist.

Abilene—*169 calories*
   3 oz. orange juice
   2 oz. peach nectar
   1 1/2 oz. dark rum

   Stir well over ice in a highball glass.

Absolut Fuzzy Navel—*139 calories*
   3 oz. fresh-squeezed orange juice.
   1 1/2 oz. Absolut Apeach vodka

   Shake and pour over ice into a tumbler.

After-Hours Coffee—*150 calories*

6 oz. hot coffee
1 oz. Rémy Martin cognac
1 tbsp. honey
Cocoa powder

Add cognac and honey to coffee. Sprinkle with cocoa powder and serve immediately.

Antifreeze—*138 calories*

1 1/2 oz. Skyy vodka
1/2 oz. Midori melon liqueur

Serve on the rocks.

Apple Cooler—*122 calories*

3 oz. apple juice
1 1/4 oz. Zaya rum

Shake well. Serve on the rocks.

Bahamas Rum Punch—*150 calories*

1 oz. Bacardi light rum
1/2 oz. Malibu coconut rum
Orange juice to taste
Pineapple juice to taste

Pour both rums in a tall glass over ice. Top with equal amounts of orange and pineapple juice.

Banana Smasher Drink—*181 calories*

1 oz. frozen orange juice concentrate
1 oz. light rum
1 tbsp. no-calorie sweetener
1 banana, sliced
3 cups crushed ice

Blend until smooth. Serve in a frosty hurricane glass.

Beefeater Berry—*110 calories*

 1 oz. Beefeater gin
 1 lime wedge, plus another for garnish
 6 oz. Ocean Spray Light cranberry juice

Muddle the gin and lime wedge in the bottom of a Collins glass. Fill the glass with ice and add cranberry juice. Tumble. Serve with a lime wedge garnish.

The Bikini—*55 calories*

 3 oz. Ocean Spray diet orange citrus juice drink
 3/4 oz. coconut-flavored rum
 Orange slice for garnish

Shake with ice and strain into a chilled glass. Garnish with the orange slice.

Blueberry Ginger Bellini—*185 calories*

1/4 cup blueberries
1 tsp. minced ginger
1 tsp. no-calorie sweetener
Juice of 1/2 lemon
1 oz. blueberry juice
2 oz. sparkling wine

Muddle blueberries with ginger, sweetener, and lemon juice. Add blueberry juice and let steep for at least 5 minutes. Strain. Top with sparkling wine.

Bourbon Cocktail—*177 calories*

2 oz. Jim Beam bourbon
2 tbsp. orange juice
1/2 cup diet tonic water
Orange peel for garnish

Fill a glass with ice. Add bourbon and orange juice. Stir in tonic water. Garnish with the orange peel.

Brave Bull—*131 calories*

1 1/2 oz. Patrón tequila
1/2 oz. Kahlúa

Serve over ice.

Burning Love—*93 calories*
1 1/2 oz. TY KU sake
Cinnamon candy hearts for garnish

Cabana Boy—*96 calories*
1 1/2 oz. TY KU liqueur
2–3 sprigs basil
2 slices ginger
2 slices seedless jalapeño pepper

Muddle all ingredients and serve over ice.

Café au Vin—*192 calories*
1 cup strong coffee, cold
2 oz. tawny port
2 tbsp. sugar
1/2 tsp. orange peel
Dash cinnamon

Blend all ingredients at high speed. Pour into a wine glass and serve.

Caipiroska—*129 calories*

1/2 lime, sliced into wedges
2 tsp. sugar
1 oz. Ultimat vodka

Place the lime wedges in the bottom of an old-fashioned glass and add sugar. Crush the sugar into the lime pulp with the end of a wooden spoon. Fill the glass with crushed ice. Pour in vodka. Stir.

Cajun Coffee—*110 calories*

1/2 cup hot coffee
1 tbsp. molasses
1 tbsp. dark rum
Whipped cream to top
Sprinkle of nutmeg

Combine the coffee and molasses in a saucepan. Heat and stir until the molasses is dissolved and the coffee is very hot, but not boiling. Pour the rum into a mug. Add the coffee mixture. Top with whipped cream and sprinkle with nutmeg.

California Lemonade—*150 calories*
2 oz. orange juice
3/4 oz. vodka
1/4 oz. cognac
1/4 oz. gin
1/4 oz. grenadine
Splash lime juice
Splash simple syrup
Fresh raspberry for garnish
Lime slice for garnish

Shake and pour into a glass over ice. Garnish with the raspberry and lime slice.

CC & Soda—*100 calories*
3 oz. club soda
1 1/2 oz. Canadian Club whisky

Charrita Margarita—*199 calories*
1 1/2 oz. Don Roberto Añejo tequila
1 1/4 oz. lime juice
1/2 oz. agave nectar
1/2 oz. orange liqueur
1/2 oz. water

Rim a margarita glass with salt. Shake with ice and pour into the glass.
Created by Junior Merino

Cherry Bomb Lite—*104 calories*
4 oz. Diet Coke
1 1/2 oz. Three Olives cherry vodka

Serve in a tall glass over ice.

Chichi—*135 calories*
1 oz. Ultimat vodka
1 tbsp. Coco López Lite cream of coconut
1 tbsp. half and half
1 tbsp. sweet and sour mix
1 tbsp. unsweetened pineapple juice
1/2 tbsp. lime juice
Maraschino cherry for garnish
Pineapple wedge for garnish

Blend vodka, cream of coconut, half and half, sweet and sour mix, pineapple juice, and lime juice. Add 1/2 cup crushed ice. Blend until smooth. Pour into a glass and fill with crushed ice. Garnish with the maraschino cherry and the pineapple wedge.

Cold Shower—*124 calories*
1 oz. Marie Brizard green crème de menthe
4 1/2 oz. soda water

Pour crème de menthe into a tall glass and top with soda water.

Cool Mist—*183 calories*
3 oz. tonic water
1 1/2 oz. Irish Mist herbal liqueur

Copenhagen—*168 calories*
6 oz. diet lemon-lime soda
1 1/2 oz. Bacardi Limón rum

Mix in a highball glass filled with ice.

Cramosa—*70 calories*
2 oz. champagne
1 oz. orange juice
1/2 oz. Ocean Spray Light cranberry juice

Pour in order listed into a champagne flute and serve chilled.

Cranberry Slush—*192 calories*
1 oz. Smirnoff vodka
1/2 oz. grapefruit juice
1/2 oz. Ocean Spray Light cranberry juice

Combine in a large freezer container. Freeze for at least 8 hours or until slushy. Spoon into a cocktail glass and serve immediately.

Crandura—*102 calories*

4 oz. Ocean Spray Light cranberry juice
1 1/2 oz. Herradura Blanco tequila
Squeeze lime
Lime wedge for garnish

Shake and strain into a rocks glass over ice. Garnish with lime wedge.

Creamsicle Punch—*81 calories*

1 oz. light orange juice
1/2 oz. Brinley Gold Shipwreck spiced rum
1/2 oz. Sobieski vodka
Diet ginger ale to top
Orange slice for garnish

Shake first three ingredients well over ice and strain into a martini glass. Top with ginger ale. Garnish with the orange slice.

Crown Fizz—*182 calories*

6 oz. diet club soda
1 1/2 oz. Crown Royal whisky
1 1/2 oz. lemon juice
4 tsp. sugar
Lemon slice for garnish

Shake with ice and serve on the rocks in a tall glass. Garnish with the lemon slice.

Cuba Libre—*193 calories*

1 lime
2 oz. Rhum Barbancourt
4 oz. diet cola

Squeeze lime into a Collins glass and then drop in the lime. Muddle. Fill the glass with ice. Add rum. Top with cola.

Cuervo Margarita—*112 calories*

3 oz. light lemonade
1 oz. Jose Cuervo Especial tequila
3/4 oz. lime juice
1/2 oz. orange liqueur
Lime wedge for garnish

Shake well with ice. Strain into an ice-filled margarita glass, or serve straight up in a cocktail glass. Garnish with a lime wedge.

Cuervo Paloma—*111 calories*

3 oz. light Ruby Red grapefruit juice
1 1/2 oz. Jose Cuervo Silver tequila
3 oz. soda water
Grapefruit peel or lime wedge for garnish

Shake first two ingredients well with ice. Strain into an ice-filled Collins glass. Top with soda water and garnish with a grapefruit peel or lime wedge.

Daiquiri—*155 calories*

2 oz. Bacardi light rum
2 oz. lemon juice
1/2 oz. water
1 tsp. no-calorie sweetener

Shake or blend with ice.

Dandy Shandy—*97 calories*

4 oz. dark stout beer
4 oz. diet ginger ale or diet ginger beer

Place dark stout beer in a serving glass. Top with ginger ale or ginger beer.

Downeaster—*138 calories*

1 oz. diet pineapple juice
1 oz. Ocean Spray Light cranberry juice
1 oz. Stolichnaya vodka
Lime wedge for garnish

Serve in an old-fashioned glass over ice. Garnish with the lime wedge.

Eco-Mojito (aka Açai Mojito)—*139 calories*

 2 oz. VeeV açaí spirit
 3/4 oz. simple syrup
 4 lime wedges
 6 mint leaves
 Club soda to top

Shake the first four ingredients well with ice and transfer to a rocks glass. Top with club soda and stir well.

Elderflower Sparklers—*54 calories*

 1 tbsp. elderflower concentrate
 1 oz. extra-dry champagne
 1 oz. seltzer
 Mint sprigs for garnish

Place elderflower concentrate in a champagne glass. Add champagne to the glass. Top off with seltzer. Garnish with mint.

Endless Summer Cocktail—*150 calories*

    2 slices cucumber
    2 slices lemon
    1 slice lime
    1/2 oz. agave nectar
    1 3/4 oz. paQui Silvera tequila
    Splash lemon-lime soda

Muddle the cucumber, lemon, and lime with the agave nectar, and then add the tequila. Serve over ice in a 12 oz. rocks glass. Top with a splash of lemon-lime soda.

Created by Santiago Santos, Beso

Espresso Nudge—*172 calories*

    1 oz. brandy
    1 oz. crème de cacao
    4 oz. hot water
    2 oz. espresso
    Light whipped cream to top

Combine brandy and crème de cacao in a 12 oz. mug. Add hot water and espresso. Top with whipped cream. Serve immediately.

Firebird—*130 calories*
  4 oz. Ocean Spray Light cranberry juice
  1 1/2 oz. Absolut Peppar vodka

  Shake with ice. Serve on the rocks.

Firefly—*132 calories*
  2 oz. grapefruit juice
  1 1/2 oz. Sobieski vodka
  Dash grenadine

Foghorn—*185 calories*
  2 oz. Magellan gin
  1/2 oz. fresh lime juice
  5 oz. diet ginger beer
  Lime wedge

  Add gin and lime juice to an ice-filled old-fashioned glass. Top with ginger beer. Stir gently. Squeeze a lime wedge over the drink and drop it in for garnish.

Fountain of Youth—*118 calories*

3 oz. pure coconut water
2 oz. VeeV açaí spirit
3/4 oz. passion fruit puree
Freshly grated orange zest for garnish

Shake well with ice and strain into an ice-filled highball glass. Garnish with orange zest.

French 75—*117 calories*

1 1/4 oz. gin
1 oz. lemon juice
1 tsp. sugar
Dry champagne to top

Place three ice cubes, gin, lemon juice, and sugar in a cocktail shaker and shake well. Strain into a champagne glass, then top with champagne.

French Connection—*150 calories*

1 oz. cognac
1 oz. Grand Marnier

Fruitie Tootie Kiss—*100 calories*

3 oz. Honest Ade Superfruit punch
1 oz. Herradura Blanco tequila
Strawberry for garnish

Serve over ice. Garnish with a strawberry.

Gibson—*157 calories*

2 oz. Beefeater gin
1/4 oz. dry vermouth
1/2 cup ice cubes
Cocktail onions for garnish

Shake first two ingredients with ice until very cold. Strain into a chilled martini glass. Garnish with cocktail onions.

Gin & Tonic—*103 calories*

3 oz. diet tonic water
1 oz. Tanqueray gin

Serve in a tall glass with ice.

Gin Buck—*178 calories*
1 1/2 oz. Magellan gin
1 tbsp. lemon juice
6 oz. diet ginger ale

Shake first two ingredients. Pour into an old-fashioned glass over ice, and top with ginger ale.

Gin Martini—*175 calories*
2 1/2 oz. Bombay gin
1/8 oz. vermouth

Shake with ice. Serve on the rocks.

Ginger Crush—*85 calories*
2 oz. diet ginger ale
1 1/2 oz. TY KU sake
Ginger snap cookie for garnish

Serve in a tall glass over ice. Garnish with a ginger snap cookie.

Grape Breeze—*119 calories*
2 oz. diet grape juice
1 oz. Absolut vodka
1/2 oz. diet pineapple juice
1/2 oz. Ocean Spray Light cranberry juice

Shake all ingredients together and strain into a glass with ice.

Grapehound—*170 calories*
6 oz. diet pink grapefruit juice
1 1/2 oz. grape vodka

Shake ingredients with ice. Serve on the rocks.

Green Tea Mojito—*69 calories*
Juice of 1/2 lime
6 large mint leaves, plus extra for garnish
1 tsp. sugar
2/3 cup brewed green tea, chilled
1 1/2 oz. white rum

Pour the lime juice into a highball glass. Add the mint and sugar and muddle them. Fill the glass with ice and add the tea and rum. Stir well. Garnish with the mint leaf.

Hair of Dragon's Breath—*130 calories*

1 oz. Absolut vodka
1/2 oz. Absolut Peppar vodka
4 oz. light V8 vegetable juice
Dash Tabasco sauce
Cilantro leaf for garnish

Fill a highball glass halfway with ice. Add in both vodkas. Fill with vegetable juice. Top with Tabasco sauce. Garnish with a cilantro leaf.

Hard Cream Soda—*128 calories*

1 oz. Smirnoff vanilla vodka
4 oz. diet cream soda

Pour vodka into a tall glass with ice. Top with diet cream soda.

Havana Beach—*120 calories*

1/2 lime
2 oz. light pineapple juice
1 oz. Bacardi white rum
1 tsp. sugar
Diet ginger ale to top
Lime slice for garnish

Quarter the lime and place it in a blender with pineapple juice, rum, and sugar. Blend until smooth. Strain into a hurricane glass. Top with ginger ale. Garnish with a lime slice.

Havana Cocktail—*79 calories*

2 oz. pineapple juice
3/4 oz. Bacardi light rum
1 tsp. lemon juice
Lemon peel for garnish

Shake with ice and strain into a glass. Garnish with the lemon peel.

Havana Delight—*196 calories*
1 1/2 oz. Coco López Lite cream of coconut
3/4 oz. Bacardi rum
1/4 oz. Kahlúa

Blend till smooth. Pour over crushed ice and serve in a margarita glass.

Hawaiian Sunset Cocktail—*178 calories*
2 1/2 oz. Ocean Spray Light cranberry juice
2 1/2 oz. orange juice
1 oz. Ultimat vodka
1 1/2 oz. soda water
Maraschino cherry for garnish

Shake cranberry juice, orange juice, and vodka in a shaker. Pour over ice in a highball glass. Top with soda water. Garnish with a maraschino cherry.

High TY-de—*110 calories*
2 oz. iced tea
1 1/2 oz. TY KU soju
3 raspberries for garnish

Shake over ice. Serve in a tall glass with ice. Garnish with the raspberries.

Honest Kiss-Tini—*100 calories*
3 oz. Honest Ade cranberry lemonade
1 oz. Herradura Blanco tequila
Dash lime juice

Serve in a tall glass with ice.

Irish Cooler—*140 calories*
6 oz. club soda
2 oz. Jameson Irish whiskey

Irish Highball—*140 calories*
4 oz. diot ginger ale
2 oz. Jameson Irish whiskey

Island Breeze—*66 calories*
2 oz. Vita Coco coconut water
1 1/2 oz. TY KU sake
Slice fresh cucumber for garnish

Shake over ice. Serve in a tall glass with ice and
garnish with the cucumber slice.

Jamaican Mule—*96 calories*

1 oz. Appleton Estate rum
Squeeze lime wedge
Diet ginger beer to top

Fill a highball glass with ice. Add rum. Squeeze the lime wedge into the rum, and top with ginger beer.

Jeremiah Sweet Tea & Light Lemonade—*123 calories*

3 oz. light lemonade
1 1/2 oz. Jeremiah Weed sweet tea flavored vodka
1/4 oz. lemon juice
3 mint leaves, plus extra for garnish
Lemon slices for garnish

Stir well with ice and strain into an ice-filled rocks or Collins glass. Garnish with lemon slices and/or mint leaves.

Kahlúa & Cognac—*155 calories*

1 oz. Kahlúa
1 oz. Rémy Martin cognac

Pour Kahlúa and cognac into a brandy snifter. Swirl gently.

Kahlúa & Iced Tea—*132 calories*

1 1/2 oz. Kahlúa
Iced tea to fill

Pour iced tea into a tall glass, then add Kahlúa.
Stir well.

Kahlúa & Soda—*135 calories*

1 1/2 oz. Kahlúa
Club soda to top
Lime wedge for garnish

Pour Kahlúa over ice in a highball glass. Top with
club soda. Stir. Garnish with a lime wedge.

Kahlúa, Rum & Soda—*164 calories*

1 1/2 oz. Kahlúa
1/2 oz. rum
Club soda to top

Pour Kahlúa and rum over ice in a tall glass. Top
with club soda.

Ketel, Cucumber, & Ginger—*127 calories*

1 1/2 oz. light lemonade
1 oz. Ketel One vodka
1/2 oz. Stirrings ginger liqueur
1/4 oz. honey syrup
2 1/4-inch cucumber rounds for garnish

Shake well with ice and strain into a well-chilled martini glass. Garnish with cucumber rounds.

Ketel One Lemon Drop—*102 calories*

2 oz. light lemonade
1 1/2 oz. Ketel One Citroen vodka
1/4 oz. lemon juice
1 packet sugar substitute
Lemon twist for garnish

Shake lemonade, vodka, and lemon juice well with ice. Strain into a well-chilled martini glass rimmed with sugar substitute. Garnish with a lemon twist.

Kickin' Carolina Tea—*125 calories*

    4 oz. diet lemon-lime soda
    1 1/2 oz. Firefly vodka
    2 tsp. light lemonade
    Lemon wedge for garnish

Put ice cubes in a glass and add ingredients in the order listed. Garnish with the lemon wedge.

Limón Mojito—*187 calories*

    1 tsp. light brown sugar
    1 lime, quartered
    8 mint leaves
    2 oz. Bacardi Limón rum
    Soda water to top
    Lemon slice for garnish
    Lime slice for garnish

Muddle the brown sugar, lime quarters, and mint in a highball glass. Fill with crushed ice and add the rum. Stir and top with soda water. Garnish with lemon and lime slices.

Low-Cal Frangelini—*155 calories*

2 oz. vanilla vodka
1/2 oz. Frangelico hazelnut liqueur
Club soda to top
Chocolate-covered espresso bean for garnish

Shake first two ingredients over ice and pour into a cold martini glass. Top with club soda. Garnish with a chocolate-covered espresso bean.

Mango Fizz—*104 calories*

4 oz. seltzer water
1 1/2 oz. Three Olives mango vodka

Serve in a tall glass with ice.

Manhattan—*170 calories*

2 oz. Maker's Mark bourbon
1/2 oz. sweet vermouth
Dash bitters
Maraschino cherry for garnish

Shake with ice until very cold, then strain into a chilled martini glass. Garnish with a cherry.

Marula Double Shot—*133 calories*

1 oz. Amarula cream liqueur
1 pinch ground ginger
1/2 tsp. strawberry preserves
1/4 oz. guava juice
Splash lime juice

Shake all ingredients except Amarula and strain into a shot glass. Pour Amarula into a separate shot glass. First shoot the Amarula, followed immediately by the strawberry spice shot.
Created by Alex Ott

Melt My Heart Mojito—*81 calories*

1 1/2 oz. TY KU liqueur
1 oz. diet lemon-lime soda
Squeeze lemon
Squeeze orange

Serve in a tall glass with ice.

Memphis Iced Tea—*70 calories*

3 oz. club soda
1 oz. Crown Royal whisky
1/2 oz. low-calorie iced tea
Lemon slice for garnish

Stir gently in a tall glass over ice. Garnish with a lemon slice.

Miami Heat Martini—*180 calories*

2 oz. Skyy vodka
1 oz. lemon juice
1/2 tsp. grenadine
1/2 tsp. superfine sugar
Maraschino cherry for garnish

Shake well with ice. Pour into a martini glass, and garnish with a maraschino cherry.

Midori Fizz—*80 calories*

1 oz. Midori melon liqueur
Top with club soda

Mix and serve over ice in a tall glass.

Midori Melonade—*80 calories*

    1 oz. Midori melon liqueur

    3 oz. Crystal Light lemonade

    Lemon wheel or wedge for garnish

Pour Midori into a tall glass over ice and top with lemonade. Stir well and garnish with a lemon wheel or wedge.

Mimosa—*113 calories*

    3 oz. champagne

    3 oz. orange juice

    Orange wedge for garnish

Fill a chilled champagne flute halfway with champagne. Top with orange juice. Garnish with an orange wedge.

Mint Cherry Jubilee—*144 calories*

    4 oz. club soda

    2 oz. Bulldog gin

    3 bing cherries for garnish

    2 mint leaves for garnish

Serve in a tall glass with ice.

Created by Raymond Bernard

Mojito—*132 calories*
   1 1/2 oz. Bacardi rum
   1/2 oz. lime juice
   2 tsp. sugar substitute
   Crushed mint to taste

   Serve in a tall glass with ice.

Mudslide—*184 calories*
   3/4 oz. Baileys Irish cream
   3/4 oz. Kahlúa
   3/4 oz. vodka

   Serve in a tall glass with ice.

Myers's Planter's Punch—*159 calories*

3 oz. orange juice
1 1/2 oz. Myers's rum
Juice from 1 lime
1 tsp. superfine sugar
Dash grenadine
Maraschino cherry for garnish
Mint sprig for garnish
Orange slice for garnish

Mix first three ingredients in a shaker. Add sugar and grenadine. Shake until frothy. Serve over shaved ice in a highball glass. Garnish with the maraschino cherry, mint sprig, and orange slice.

No-Guilt Margarita—*120 calories*

4 oz. seltzer water
1 oz. fresh-squeezed lime juice
1 1/2 oz. 1800 tequila
2 packets no-calorie sweetener

Serve in a tall glass with ice.

Old-Fashioned—*180 calories*

1 tsp. sugar
Dash bitters
Orange slice
2 oz. bourbon
1/2 cup ice cubes
Maraschino cherry for garnish

In a rocks glass combine sugar, bitters, and an orange slice. Crush with the back of a spoon. Add bourbon and 1/2 cup ice cubes. Garnish with a maraschino cherry.

Orange You Nice—*130 calories*

4 oz. Ocean Spray Light cranberry juice
1 1/2 oz. Sobieski orange vodka

Shake with ice. Serve up or on the rocks.

Oyster Shooter—*104 calories*

1 small freshly shucked raw oyster with its juice
1 oz. ice-cold vodka
Dash Tabasco sauce
Squeeze fresh lemon juice

Place the oyster and its juice in the bottom of a chilled martini or shot glass. Pour in the vodka, then add Tabasco sauce and lemon juice. Drink as a shot, allowing oyster to slide down your throat. Try not to chew.

Paloma—*150 calories*

5 oz. diet grapefruit soda
2 oz. Herradura tequila
1 oz. lemon juice
Pinch salt

Shake and strain into a rocks glass with ice.

Parrot Bay Breeze—*176 calories*

  3 oz. pineapple juice
  2 oz. Ocean Spray Light cranberry juice
  1 1/2 oz. Captain Morgan Parrot Bay coconut rum

Combine ingredients in a highball glass over crushed ice. Stir well and serve.

Peppy Tomato Sipper—*105 calories*

  4 oz. low-sodium V8 vegetable juice
  1 oz. vodka
  1 tbsp. lime juice
  1/2 tsp. Worcestershire sauce
  1/4 tsp. horseradish
  Tabasco sauce to taste
  Celery sticks for garnish

Combine ingredients in a small pitcher, then pour mixture over ice. Garnish with celery sticks.

Piña Colada—*168 calories*

2 oz. unsweetened pineapple juice
1 oz. Coco López cream of coconut
1 oz. dark rum
Maraschino cherry for garnish
Pineapple wedge for garnish

Blend with ice until smooth. Serve in a tall glass
with a maraschino cherry and a pineapple wedge
for garnish.

Piña Fizz—*135 calories*

1 1/2 oz. Artá Silver tequila
2 oz. hibiscus juice
1/2 oz. mango puree
1/4 oz. agave nectar
Lime juice to taste
Soda water to top

Build ingredients in a mixing glass, except for
soda water. Add ice, shake, strain into a tall
Collins glass, and top with soda water.

Piñata—*173 calories*

4 oz. pineapple juice
1 1/2 oz. Jose Cuervo Gold tequila

Serve in a tall glass.

Pineapple Greyhound—*114 calories*

1 1/2 oz. diet pink grapefruit juice
1 oz. pineapple juice
1 oz. Teton Glacier potato vodka
Grapefruit slice for garnish

Shake well with ice and serve on the rocks.
Garnish with a grapefruit slice.

Pink Gin (aka Gin & Bitters)—*142 calories*

2 oz. Tanqueray gin
Dash Angostura bitters

Rinse a chilled glass with bitters. Add ice and gin.

Pomegranate-Açai Lemonade—*100 calories*

2 oz. VeeV açaí spirit
Sugar-free lemonade to fill
1/4 oz. POM Wonderful pomegranate juice
2 lemon wheel slices

Add VeeV açaí spirit to a highball glass and fill it with sugar-free lemonade. Top with pomegranate juice and float the lemon wheels on top.

Pomegranate Collins—*100 calories*

3/4 oz. fresh lemon juice
1/2 oz. agave nectar
1 oz. Bombay Sapphire gin
Club soda to top
3 pomegranate seeds for garnish
Lemon wedge for garnish

Lightly muddle the lemon juice and nectar. Add gin, shake, and pour into an Ice-filled highball glass. Top with club soda. Garnish with the pomegranate seeds and lemon wedge.

Prairie Fire—*145 calories*
  2 oz. Patrón tequila
  2–3 drops Tabasco sauce

Red Berry Burst—*180 calories*
  1 oz. fresh lemon juice
  1 oz. Monin pomegranate syrup
  3/4 oz. Stolichnaya vodka
  3/4 oz. Stolichnaya Razberi vodka
  Blackberry for garnish
  Lemon wedge for garnish

  Shake well. Serve over ice in a rocks glass. Garnish
  with a blackberry and a lemon wedge.

Red Buffalo—*120 calories*
  1 oz. Buffalo Trace bourbon
  1 oz. Dubonnet Red
  1 oz. Ocean Spray Light cranberry juice
  Orange twist for garnish

  Shake well with ice and strain into a cocktail glass.
  Garnish with an orange twist.

Red Eye—*163 calories*

2 oz. tomato juice
12 oz. light beer
Seasoning salt
Lime twist
Green olives for garnish

Pour tomato juice and then beer into a chilled mug. Throw in a pinch of salt and a twist of lime. Garnish with olives and serve.

Red Rooster—*95 calories*

2 oz. Ocean Spray Light cranberry juice
1 oz. vodka
Fresh cranberries for garnish
Lemon slice for garnish

Stir and pour into a glass over ice. Garnish with the cranberries and lemon slice.

Refreshing Lemonade—*140 calories*

4 oz. frozen light lemonade, prepared
1 oz. Grey Goose vodka

Pour vodka and lemonade into a blender and fill it with ice. Puree and serve.

The Ritual—*34 calories*
1 shot Xante *(cognac liqueur with notes of spicy vanilla and pear)*

Serve over ice.

Rob Roy—*150 calories*
2 oz. Dewar's scotch whisky
1/4 oz. sweet or dry vermouth

Stir over ice and strain. Serve straight up or on the rocks.

Rose's Cocktail Infusions Cosmopolitan Light—*115 calories*
2 oz. Rose's Cocktail Infusions Cosmopolitan Light mix
1 oz. Smirnoff vodka

Shake with 1/2 cup of ice in a cocktail shaker and strain into a martini glass.

Ruby Red Sea Breeze—*100 calories*

2 oz. light Ruby Red grapefruit juice
2 oz. Ocean Spray Light cranberry juice
1 oz. Teton Glacier potato vodka

Stir. Serve in a tall glass with ice.

Rum Punch Painkiller—*194 calories*

1 oz. Coco López Lite cream of coconut
1 oz. orange juice
1 oz. pineapple juice
1 oz. spiced rum

Mix well. Serve in a tall glass on the rocks.

Rum Refresher—*105 calories*

1 oz. Jamaican dark rum
6 tbsp. fresh orange juice
6 tbsp. strong tea, chilled
Sugar to taste
Orange slice for garnish
Mint leaves or sprig for garnish

In a highball glass filled halfway with ice, combine rum, orange juice, and tea. Stir. Add sugar to taste. Garnish with the orange slice and mint.

Rum Relaxation—*149 calories*

1 1/2 oz. Bacardi light rum
1 oz. pineapple juice
1/2 oz. grenadine
Lemon-lime soda to top
Maraschino cherry for garnish
Orange slice for garnish

Shake the first three ingredients well with ice. Pour into a hurricane glass and top with lemon-lime soda. Garnish with the cherry and orange slice.

Russian Spring—*140 calories*

1 oz. Russian Standard vodka
1/2 oz. DeKuyper green crème de menthe
1 oz. apple juice
2 1/2 oz. soda water
Mint sprig for garnish

Shake the first three ingredients with ice. Strain into a highball glass filled halfway with cubed ice. Add soda water and garnish with the mint sprig.

Sake Martini—*184 calories*

2 oz. Skyy vodka
1 tsp. sake
Cucumber slice for garnish

Shake vodka and sake well. Pour into a martini glass over ice and garnish with the cucumber slice.

Salty Chihuahua—*188 calories*

1 oz. Jose Cuervo Gold tequila
1/2 oz. Cointreau
2 oz. grapefruit juice
Grapefruit slice for garnish
Coarse salt to rim glass

Wet the rim of a glass and coat it with coarse salt. Add ice. Pour the tequila and Cointreau into the glass. Top with grapefruit juice and stir. Garnish with a slice of grapefruit.

Salty Dog—*145 calories*

3 oz. grapefruit juice
1 1/2 oz. gin or vodka

Mix with ice and pour into a salt-rimmed glass.

Sand Trap—*140 calories*

2 oz. pineapple juice
1 1/2 oz. Sobieski orange vodka

Serve over ice.

Screaming Orange Soda—*147 calories*

1 oz. orange juice
1 oz. vodka
1 tbsp. sugar
3/4 tsp. vanilla extract

Blend with 1 cup of ice for 30 seconds on high.
Serve in a frosty Collins glass.

Screwdriver—*145 calories*

3 oz. orange juice
1 1/2 oz. Smirnoff vodka

Serve over ice.

Sea Breeze—*140 calories*
1 oz. light grapefruit juice
1 oz. Ocean Spray Light cranberry juice
1 oz. Sobieski vodka
1 lime wedge

Put all ingredients in a glass and stir well. Serve over crushed ice. Garnish with lime wedge.

Seven Skinny—*140 calories*
3 oz. diet 7-Up
2 oz. Seagram's 7 whisky

Skinny Caipi Cola—*99 calories*
6 oz. diet cola
1 1/2 oz. Leblon cachaça
Lime wedge for garnish

Stir in a highball glass over ice. Garnish with a lime wedge.

Slim Gin—*100 calories*
1 1/2 oz. Tanqueray gin
Diet soda to fill

Pour into a 6 oz. Collins glass. Fill with your favorite diet soda.

Smirnoff Cosmopolitan—*110 calories*

1 oz. orange liqueur
1 oz. Smirnoff vodka
1 1/2 oz. light cranberry juice
1/4 oz. lime juice
Lime wedge for garnish

Shake well with ice and strain into a well-chilled martini glass. Garnish with a lime wedge.

Sour Apple Martini—*160 calories*

2 1/2 oz. sour mix
3/4 oz. DeKuyper Sour Apple liqueur
3/4 oz. vodka

Serve in a tall glass with ice.

Sparkling Summer Spritzer—*103 calories*

4 oz. white wine
4 oz. club soda
1/4 lemon, halved

Fill a highball glass with ice and pour wine half-way. Top with club soda. Squeeze in the juice from one section of lemon. Garnish with the other section of lemon.

Spicy Lust—143 calories
1 oz. Smirnoff vodka
1 tsp. Tabasco sauce
1 pickled jalapeño for garnish

In a cocktail shaker, add a scoop of crushed ice, vodka, and Tabasco sauce. Shake well. Strain into a well-chilled martini glass. Garnish with a jalapeño pepper.

Spike—150 calories
4 oz. grapefruit juice
1 1/2 oz. Jose Cuervo Gold tequila

Combine in a highball glass.

Spritzer—60 calories
3 oz. white wine
Club soda to top

Pour white wine into a 6 oz. wine glass filled with ice. Top with club soda.

Stinger—*180 calories*

2 oz. Rémy Martin cognac
1/4 oz. DeKuyper white crème de menthe

Shake with ice. Pour into a chilled martini glass.

Stoli Lemonade—*110 calories*

1 1/2 oz. fresh-squeezed lemon juice
1 1/2 oz. Monin sugar-free simple syrup
1 1/2 oz. Stolichnaya vodka
Lemon wedge for garnish

Shake and serve over ice in a rocks glass. Garnish with a lemon wedge.

Stoli Raspberry Lemonade—*110 calories*

1 oz. fresh lemon juice
1 oz. Monin sugar-free simple syrup
1 1/2 oz. Stolichnaya *(or Stolichnaya Razberi)* vodka
3 raspberries
Lemon wedge for garnish

Combine ingredients and shake well *(no need to muddle raspberries)*. Pour ingredients straight into a rocks glass. Garnish with a raspberry and a lemon wedge.

Strawberry Basil Lemonade—*192 calories*

    1 1/2 oz. strawberry vodka
    1 oz. pureed strawberry
    5/8 cup light lemonade
    3 large basil leaves

Mix vodka and strawberry puree in a martini shaker. Add ice and shake well. Pour into a tall glass. Fill with lemonade. Add basil leaves and serve.

Strawberry-Coconut Daiquiri—*112 calories*

    1/4 cup chopped fresh or frozen strawberries
    1/2 tsp. sugar
    1/4 tsp. lime juice
    3 cups ice cubes
    1 oz. Malibu rum

Blend strawberries, sugar, and lime juice until smooth. Add ice cubes and rum. Blend until frothy.

Strawberry-Mango Lemonade—*193 calories*

 2 oz. Dole Chef-Ready Cuts diced strawberries
 2 oz. Dole Chef-Ready Cuts mango cubes
 1 1/4 oz. lime rum
 2 oz. sour mix
 Squeeze lemon juice
 1 oz. lemon-lime soda
 Lemon corkscrew for garnish

Muddle strawberries and mango cubes in a shaker. Combine rum, fresh sour, and lemon juice in the shaker with ice. Shake vigorously then strain into a glass with ice. Top with soda. Garnish with a lemon corkscrew.

Strawberry Soju Sunshine—*135 calories*

 1 1/2 oz. TY KU soju
 3 fresh strawberries
 Fresh yuzu citrus to fill

Serve in a tall glass with ice. Fill with fresh yuzu citrus.

Summer Watermelon Mojito—*141 calories*

5 chopped mint leaves
1/4 tsp. no-calorie sweetener
1/4 oz. fresh lime juice, separated
1 1/2 oz. light rum
6 oz. pureed seedless watermelon

In the bottom of a large shaker, muddle the mint, sweetener, and 1/8 oz. lime juice. Fill the shaker with ice. Add rum, watermelon puree, and remaining lime juice. Shake well. Strain into an old-fashioned glass over ice.

Sunburn Cooler—*185 calories*

6 raspberries
4 slices green bell pepper
1 1/2 oz. TY KU liqueur
1/2 oz. lime juice
1/4 oz. ginger liqueur

Muddle raspberries and pepper. Add TY KU liqueur, lime juice, and ginger liqueur. Serve over ice.

Sunkist Blushing Grapefruit
Cosmo—*167 calories*

1 1/2 oz. vodka
1/2 oz. Grand Marnier
2 oz. fresh-squeezed Sunkist red grapefruit juice
Sugar to rim glass
Grapefruit twist for garnish

Fill a shaker with ice and add vodka, Grand Marnier, and grapefruit juice. Cover and shake well. Coat the rim of a martini glass with sugar. Strain the drink into the glass. Garnish with a grapefruit twist.

Sunkist Lemon Drop—*195 calories*

2 oz. citrus vodka
1/2 oz. limoncello liqueur
1/4 oz. Sunkist lemon juice
1 tsp. sugar, plus more to rim glass
Sunkist lemon juice ice cubes
Lemon twist for garnish

Fill a shaker with lemon juice ice cubes. *(In an ice tray, fill with ¾ lemon juice and ¼ water. Freeze.)* Add vodka, limoncello, lemon juice, and sugar. Cover and shake well. Pour into a sugar-rimmed martini glass and garnish with a lemon twist.

Sunkist Slightly Orange Martini— *135 calories*

Sunkist orange juice ice cubes
2 oz. Sobieski orange vodka
1/2 oz. Sunkist fresh-squeezed orange juice
Orange twist for garnish

Fill a shaker with orange juice ice cubes. *(In an ice tray, fill with ¾ orange juice and ¼ water. Freeze.)* Add vodka and orange juice, then cover and shake well. Strain into a chilled martini glass and garnish with an orange twist.

Sunny-Tini—*100 calories*

1 1/2 oz. chilled Sobieski vodka
Sugar to rim glass
Orange slice for garnish

Serve in a chilled, sugar-rimmed glass with an orange slice.

Sunshine in a Glass—*130 calories*

2 oz. orange juice
1 1/2 oz. Sobieski orange vodka
Orange slice for garnish

Serve in a tall glass with an orange slice.

'Ti Punch—*120 calories*

3 tbsp. white rum
1 tsp. lime juice
1 1/2 tsp. brown sugar

Add rum and lime juice to a wine glass over ice
cubes. Add brown sugar and stir to mix well.

Tropicana Cocktail—*170 calories*

2 oz. grapefruit juice
2 oz. pineapple juice
1 1/4 oz. Bacardi light rum
Pineapple ring for garnish

Shake with ice. Serve over ice with a ring of
pineapple.

Vanilla Cape Codder—*150 calories*

3 oz. Ocean Spray Light cranberry juice
1 1/2 oz. vanilla vodka

Serve over ice.

Vodka Gimlet—*145 calories*
  2 oz. Skyy vodka
  1/4 oz. lime juice

  Shake well. Serve in a chilled martini glass.

Vodka Martini—*175 calories*
  2 1/2 oz. Teton Glacier potato vodka
  1/8 oz. vermouth

  Shake with ice. Serve on the rocks.

Vodka Tonic—*128 calories*
  3 oz. tonic water
  1 1/2 oz. 360 vodka

Wake Me Up Martini—*130 calories*
  1 oz. citrus vodka
  1 oz. grapefruit juice
  1 oz. orange juice

  Shake and strain into a martini glass.

White Chocolate Irish Coffee—*174 calories*

3/4 cup hot coffee
3/4 oz. Baileys Irish Cream
3/4 oz. Irish whiskey
1/2 oz. white crème de cacao

Pour all ingredients into a mug. Stir and serve.

Wild Irish Rose—*185 calories*

1 1/2 oz. Tullamore Dew Irish whiskey
3/4 oz. lemon juice
1/2 oz. grenadine
2 oz. sparkling soda water
Maraschino cherry for garnish

Fill an old-fashioned glass 3/4 full with ice. Pour whiskey, lemon juice, and grenadine over the ice. Top with sparkling soda water. Stir gently. Garnish with a maraschino cherry.

Will You Be My TY-Tini?—*94 calories*

1 1/2 oz. TY KU liqueur
1 1/2 oz. TY KU soju
Squeeze lime
Splash diet lemon-lime soda

Serve in a tall glass with ice.

World's Freshest Margarita—*160 calories*
2 oz. Milagro tequila
1/4 tbsp. agave nectar
1 oz. fresh lime juice
Lime wheel for garnish

Shake with ice. Strain over fresh ice in a rocks glass and garnish with a lime wheel.

Zen Cooler—*150 calories*
1 oz. Zen green tea liqueur
Fresca to top

Mix and serve over ice in a tall glass.

Zen Iced Tea—*150 calories*
1 oz. Zen green tea liqueur
Crystal Light iced tea to top
Lemon wedge for garnish

Mix and serve over ice in a tall glass. Garnish with a lemon wedge.

Part III
Skinny Nonalcoholic Drinks

Skipping the alcohol doesn't have to
mean skipping the fun or flavor. Tasty,
low-calorie nonalcoholic options will keep
you refreshed all night long so you can
wake up to a guilt-free morning.

Cherry Sparkle—*107 calories*

8 oz. sparkling water
2 tbsp. pure black cherry juice extract
Maraschino cherry for garnish
Orange, lemon, or lime slice for garnish

Add sparkling water to a glass and mix in the cherry juice extract. Garnish with a slice of orange, lemon, or lime and a cherry.

Coke and Drops—*106 calories*

1 cup Coca-Cola
7 drops lemon juice
Lemon slice for garnish

Pour the Coca-Cola in a glass and add 7 drops of lemon juice. Garnish with the lemon slice.

Cranberry Burst—*160 calories*

6 oz. Ocean Spray Light cranberry juice with calcium
2 oz. orange juice
2 oz. ginger ale or diet ginger ale
Orange slice for garnish

Pour into a glass with ice. Garnish with the orange slice.

Cranberry Kiss—*112 calories*

6 oz. Ocean Spray Light cranberry juice
1 oz. orange juice
Club soda
Orange wedge for garnish

Pour cranberry juice and orange juice into a glass
with ice. Top with club soda. Garnish with the
orange wedge.

Delightful Cranberry
Lemonade—*178 calories*

8 oz. Ocean Spray Light cranberry juice
4 oz. lemonade
Lemon slice for garnish

Pour into a large glass filled with ice. Garnish with
the lemon slice.

Evil Princess—*157 calories*

2 oz. grape juice
1 oz. apple juice
1 oz. grenadine
1 tbsp. vanilla syrup
1 tbsp. lemon juice
Lime slice for garnish

Pour over ice, stir, and garnish with a lime slice.

Lime Tonic—*65 calories*

6 oz. tonic water
1 oz. lime juice
Lime wedge for garnish

Pour tonic water and lime juice into a highball glass almost filled with ice cubes. Stir well. Garnish with a lime wedge.

Piña Colada Cooler—*165 calories*

4 oz. sparkling water
3 oz. pineapple juice
1 tbsp. Coco Lopez light cream of coconut *(found in the drink mixers section of many supermarkets)*

Pour ingredients over ice and stir.

Raspberry Cranberry Lemon
Berry Squeeze—*134 calories*

6 oz. Ocean Spray Light cran-raspberry juice
Squeeze lemon
6 oz. club soda
Lemon twist for garnish

Combine cran-raspberry juice and lemon juice in a tall glass with ice. Top with club soda and stir gently. Garnish with a twist of lemon.

Rose's Cosmopolitan Light
Spritzer—*45 calories*

2 oz. Rose's Cocktail Infusions cosmopolitan light
2 oz. Diet 7-Up
1/2 cup ice

Combine and serve over ice.

Rose's Cosmo Spritzer—*45 calories*

3 oz. Canada Dry diet ginger ale
2 oz. Rose's Cocktail Infusions cosmopolitan light
1/2 cup ice

Combine and serve over ice.

Rose's Cranappletini—*143 calories*

3/4 oz. Rose's Cocktail Infusions sour apple
3/4 oz. Rose's Cocktail Infusions cosmopolitan
   light
1/2 cup ice

Shake with ice and strain into martini glass.

Rose's Purple Gecko Martini—*143 calories*

3/4 oz. Rose's Cocktail Infusions blue raspberry
3/4 oz. Rose's Cocktail Infusions cosmopolitan
   light
1/2 cup ice

Shake with ice and strain into martini glass.

Rose's Sunset Martini—*109 calories*

2 oz. Rose's Cocktail Infusions cosmopolitan light
1/2 cup ice

Shake with ice and strain into martini glass.

Rose's Tropical Fruit Twist Light Martini-- *109 calories*

2 oz. Rose's Cocktail Infusions tropical fruit twist light

1/2 cup ice

Shake with ice and strain into martini glass.

Rose's Tropical Fruit Twist Light Spritzer--*45 calories*

2 oz. Rose's Cocktail Infusions tropical fruit twist light

2 oz. Diet 7-Up

1/2 cup ice

Combine and serve over ice.

Summer Rain—*178 calories*

  2 oz. orange sherbet

  1 oz. raspberry purée

  1 oz. grapefruit juice, plus a grapefruit wedge
  for garnish

  1 oz. pineapple juice, plus a pineapple wedge
  for garnish

  1 oz. lemonade

Blend the first four ingredients briefly with half a glassful of crushed ice and pour into a highball glass. Add lemonade and garnish with fruit.

Summer Sunshine Cocktail—*74 calories*

  3 oz. lemon juice

  2 oz. orange juice

  1 oz. pineapple juice

  1 oz. lime juice

  Lemon slice for garnish *(optional)*

  Lime slice for garnish *(optional)*

Pour over ice and stir. Add a straw *(optional, but if you do, you might want it to be a yellow one)* and garnish with a lemon or lime slice—or both—and enjoy the shocking sour taste!

Sunkist Hemingway's
Virgin Daiquiri—*154 calories*

8 oz. Sunkist grapefruit juice

1/2 oz. fresh lime juice

1/2 oz. Maraschino cherry juice

1 tsp. sugar *(optional)*

1 cup ice

Maraschino cherry for garnish

Sunkist grapefruit wedge for garnish

Add grapefruit juice, lime juice, maraschino cherry juice, sugar *(if desired)*, and ice to a blender. Blend until almost smooth. Pour into a cocktail glass. Garnish with a cherry and grapefruit wedge held by an umbrella.

Sunkist Lemon Daisy—*149 calories*

3/4 oz. fresh lemon juice

1/2 oz. grenadine syrup

1/2 oz. simple syrup

1/2 oz. 7-Up soda

1/2 oz. soda water

Stir the lemon juice, grenadine, and simple syrup together in a white wine glass. Add ice and top with equal parts 7-Up and soda water.

Virgin Flamingo Cocktail—*104 calories*

4 oz. Ocean Spray Light cranberry juice
2 oz. pineapple juice
1/2 oz. lemon juice
2 oz. club soda
Lime wedge for garnish

Pour the cranberry juice, pineapple juice, and lemon juice into a cocktail shaker half-filled with ice cubes. Shake well and strain into a highball glass. Top with the club soda and stir well. Garnish with a lime wedge.

Virgin Manhattan—*68 calories*

1/4 cup Ocean Spray Light cranberry juice
1/4 cup orange juice
1/2 tsp. Maraschino cherry juice
1/4 tsp. lemon juice
1/4 tsp. orange zest
Maraschino cherry for garnish

Shake ingredients with ice. Strain into a chilled cocktail glass or on the rocks in an old-fashioned glass. Garnish with a maraschino cherry.

Virgin Mimosa—*116 calories*

1 cup granulated sugar
1/4 cup sparkling apple cider
1/4 cup orange juice
Juice of 1/2 lemon
Lemon zest for garnish *(optional)*

Pour a small amount of sugar onto a saucer. Wet the rim of a champagne glass and press the glass, upside down, into the sugar, "frosting" the rim. Pour in cider, orange juice, and lemon juice. Garnish with lemon zest, if desired.

Virgin Smoothie—*116 calories*

2 cups honeydew melon, chopped
1 small apple, with skin, chopped
1/2 cup kiwi
2 tbsp. lemon juice
1 cup ice cubes

Mix the ingredients in a blender until they become slushy and pour into glasses.

Warm Cranberry Apple
Wassail—*140 calories*

 1 48-oz. bottle *(or 6 cups)* Ocean Spray Light
   cranberry juice
 2 cups apple juice
 4 3-in. cinnamon sticks
 1 tsp. whole allspice
 1/4 tsp. ginger
 Orange slices for garnish
 Whole cloves for garnish

Combine ingredients in a large saucepan. Heat
to boiling, then reduce heat and simmer for 10
minutes. Strain punch to remove spices. Pour
into a heat-proof punch bowl or individual serving
mugs. Garnish with orange slices studded with
cloves, if desired.

Makes about 12 6-oz. servings.

Warm Winter White Wassail—*139 calories*

1 64-oz. bottle Ocean Spray white cranberry juice
4 3-in. cinnamon sticks, plus 6 more for garnish
1/4 tsp. ground ginger
6 tsp. butter, softened
6 tsp. brown sugar
3 oz. almond liqueur *(optional)*

Combine juice, 4 cinnamon sticks, and ginger in a large saucepan. Heat to boiling, then reduce heat and simmer for 10 minutes.

Put 1 tsp. each of butter and brown sugar in 6 large mugs. Pour the hot juice mixture into each mug. Stir gently. Add 1/2 oz. almond liqueur to each mug, if desired. Garnish with the remaining cinnamon sticks.

Makes 6 servings.

Wavebender—*83 calories*

1 oz. orange juice
1/2 oz. lemon juice
1 tsp. grenadine
5 oz. ginger ale

Pour the orange juice, lemon juice, and grenadine into a cocktail shaker half-filled with ice cubes. Shake well and strain into a highball glass almost filled with ice cubes. Top with ginger ale and stir well.

Websites

www.bartender.com

www.mixologist.com

www.usbartender.com

www.caloriecount.about.com

www.calorieking.com

www.thedailyplate.com

www.thecaloriecounter.com

www.dietitian.com

www.my-calorie-counter.com

www.calorielab.com

www.bmi-calculator.net

www.3fatchicks.com

www.caloriecountercharts.com

www.caloriecountingtips.com

www.beer100.com/beercalories

www.trytyku.com

www.sunkistfs.com/equipment
www.corzo.com
www.midori-world.com
www.herradura.com
www.bulldoggin.com
www.1800tequila.com
www.dole.com
www.oceanspray.com
www.amarula.com
www.tequiladonroberto.com
www.artatequila.com
www.haamoniismooth.com
www.vodkasobieski.com

Your Skinny Recipes

Drink Index

Alcohol Index

𝒲

𝒳

About the Authors

Jaclyn Wilson Foley has been the editor of *Bartender Magazine* for more than thirty years. She is a graduate of Rosemont College in Pennsylvania. Jackie is the author of *Girls' Night*, which features more than a thousand recipes for going out, staying in, and having fun. She resides in Basking Ridge, New Jersey, with her husband, the omnicogniscient Ray Foley, founder of *Bartender Magazine*, and their son, Ryan Peter.